Ketogenic Cooking

Ketogenic Cooking With Your Instant Pot

LELA GIBSON

CONTENTS

Introduction — 5

1 Ketogenic Cooking: Getting Started — 8

2 Instant Pot Cooking Tips — 11

3 Breakfast Recipes — 13

4 Lunch Recipes — 23

5 Dinner Recipes — 32

6 Desserts — 40

7 I need your help... — 52

Introduction

I want to thank you and congratulate you for buying the book, "Ketogenic Cooking".

This book contains proven steps and strategies on how to cook ketogenic recipes with your instant pot.

If you have been trying to lose weight for some time, you are likely to have come across the ketogenic diet. This diet is effective in not only weight loss but also reversing type 2 diabetes, improving mental health among other things. Despite all the amazing benefits this diet enables you to enjoy, some people get bored preparing the same ketogenic recipes.

However, I have good news that will revolutionize your cooking. Are you aware that you can prepare tasty ketogenic recipes using an instant pot? If you think that just because you adopted the ketogenic diet, you will have to get rid of using your instant pot, think again. This book has tasty ketogenic recipes that you can prepare in your instant pot.

Thanks again for buying this book, I hope you enjoy it!

against the publisher for any reparation, damages, or monetary loss due to the information herein, either directly or indirectly.

Respective authors own all copyrights not held by the publisher.

The information herein is offered for informational purposes solely, and is universal as so. The presentation of the information is without contract or any type of guarantee assurance.

The trademarks that are used are without any consent, and the publication of the trademark is without permission or backing by the trademark owner. All trademarks and brands within this book are for clarifying purposes only and are the owned by the owners themselves, not affiliated with this document.

Ketogenic Cooking: Getting Started

The ketogenic diet is a high fat low carb diet designed to allow the body enter a state of ketosis. In this state, your body relies on fat for energy.

Usually, our bodies prefer carbohydrates for energy. Therefore, when you take a high carb meal, the carbohydrates are converted to glucose and the body uses the glucose for energy. Any excess glucose is converted to fat for storage. The more carbohydrates you take, the more any excess are converted to fat for storage. Over time, as your increase your carbohydrate intake, you also increase your fat storage, which only leads to weight gain. With the Ketogenic diet, you reduce your carbohydrate intake, which makes your body look for alternative sources of energy; hence, turning to burning fat for energy.

Adopting the ketogenic diet entails following some rules with regards to the quantities of your macronutrients, which include:

Fats - Fats make the ketogenic diet the success that it is. If you don't consume enough fats, you might as well stop following the diet. This is because you need to get 70% of your daily calories from fat.

Proteins – Get 20% of your daily calories from protein.

Avoid eating too much protein since excess proteins can be converted to glucose. This is done via gluconeogenesis. If your protein intake is too much, you risk getting out of ketosis, as your body will have all the glucose it needs and it won't need to burn fat for energy.

Carbohydrates - Carbohydrates have little room in the ketogenic diet. Eat only 50g or 20-25g net carbs each day.

It is important to note that just because you are following the ketogenic diet that your diet will be boring. Actually, this is quite the contrary. Modern appliances and a variety of keto recipes can enable you to enjoy ketogenic recipes for quite some time. One such amazing appliance is the Instant Pot. This top of the range electric pressure cooker comes with several benefits. These include:

Multi-use

You can use the instant pot as a steamer, a sauté pan, a rice cooker and even a slow-cooker. You can also bake in it if you want. If you want to get rid of other appliances and still have various options when cooking, the Instant Pot would be the appliance you'd want to keep. In addition, it doesn't take up a lot of space nor does it heat up the kitchen or make a lot of noise while cooking.

Programmable

We cannot talk about the Instant Pot without mentioning that it is programmable. You can program your Instant Pot 24-hours in advance, if you wish. This function allows you to place your food in the Instant Pot and go about your day without hurrying back to start preparing food. Once it reaches the time you had programmed, your Instant Pot will start doing its work. Thus, by the time you go back home, you'll have a hot freshly cooked meal waiting for you.

Timesaving

The Instant Pot lets you cook meals that would have taken 6-8 hours in a slow cooker in just an hour or even less time. Foods such as a roast can take less than 50 minutes to cook. This gives you more options even if you don't have a lot of time to wait around for meals.

Easy to clean

The Instant Pot makes cleaning easier since its cooking bowl is made of stainless steel; you can easily clean the appliance by hand or place it in the dishwasher. Further, you do not need to scrub it thoroughly. In fact, you should make a habit of cleaning it gently with some soap and warm water. Clean your Instant Pot as soon as you finish cooking. This way, it will be ready when you need to use it again.

Instant Pot Cooking Tips

To make the best use of your instant pot, follow the below tips:

Add some liquid

You need to remember that the Instant Pot is still a pressure cooker. You need to pressurize it for it to work properly. This is why you should add about 1/2-1 cup of liquid in the pot whenever you are cooking. Water or broth works to bring your Instant Pot to pressure to do its work.

Set the pressure valve to sealing

One important thing you need to remember when using the Instant Pot is to make sure the pressure valve is always turned to sealing as you cook. This will allow the Instant Pot to come to pressure to begin the cooking process. If you forget to seal the valve, you'll start hearing a whistling sound. If you do so, simply turn it, as this will allow the pot to come to pressure.

Use the pot-in-pot cooking method

The pot-in-pot method makes the Instant Pot a handy appliance to have in your kitchen. This method allows you to cook several dishes at the same time without mixing them. You can place the first dish at the bottom of the inner pot and then place the steamer rack inside. This will allow you to place another bowl or dish on top. Thus, by the end of the cooking time, you'll have two separate meal. You can even have 3 separate meals if the space in your Instant Pot allows it!

Use oven safe containers

Over safe containers are the best for use when cooking in your Instant Pot, since other containers may end up cracking. You can look for several circular containers, as they fit better inside your Instant Pot. Also, look for oven safe lids as they are useful when you don't want water to seep into your food. Oven safe containers can also come in handy when you want to use the pot-in-pot cooking method. Stainless steel bowls are especially great for this cooking method as they can transfer the heat fast.

You should also make use of your trivet, as this will allow you to bake various things by placing water at the bottom of your Instant Pot and then placing your food on top of the trivet in an oven safe container.

In the following chapters, we will look at ketogenic recipes you can make in your instant pot. Let us get started with breakfast recipes.

Breakfast Recipes

Egg Bake

Servings: 4

Ingredients

1/2 teaspoon pepper

1 teaspoon kosher salt

1/2 cup shredded cheddar cheese

1/4 cup milk

6 eggs

2 cups frozen hash browns

6 slices bacon, chopped

Optional add-ins: green onions, mushrooms, spinach, red pepper, onion

Directions

Slice bacon into bite-size pieces and sauté until crispy. Add any vegetables you want and then sauté for 3 more minutes or until tender. Add frozen hash browns and cook for 2 minutes ensuring you stir frequently.

Grease an ovenproof container, making sure that it fits into your Instant Pot.

In a bowl, whisk together shredded cheese, milk, eggs, salt and pepper and then add the vegetables and bacon. Pour the mixture into the prepared container.

Add 1 1/2 cups of water into the Instant Pot and then place the trivet inside. Place the container on top and lock the lid.

Cook for 10 minutes at high pressure. Once done, do a quick release.

Use a spatula to loosen the edges and then dump the cheesy egg bake on a plate.

Serve with extra shredded cheese and green onions if you wish.

Enjoy.

Nutritional information per serving: calories 354, fat 23.7g, carbs 16.4g, protein 18g

Keto Egg Cups

Servings: 4

Ingredients

2 tablespoons chopped cilantro or herb of choice

Salt and pepper to taste

1/4 cup half and half

1/2 cup shredded sharp cheddar cheese

1 cup diced vegetables - you can use onions, mushrooms and bell peppers

4 eggs

1/2 cup shredded cheese of choice - for finishing

Directions

In a bowl, mix the vegetables, half-and-half, eggs, cheese, salt and pepper and then add chopped cilantro if you wish.

Pour the mixture into 4 1/ pint jar containers and loosely cover them with lids in order to prevent the water from seeping in. You should ensure that the containers are oven safe.

Add 2 cups of water inside the Instant Pot and then put the trivet inside. Arrange the jars on top of the trivet. Cook at high pressure for 5 minutes and then do a quick release.

Spread the left over 1/2 cup of cheese on top of the portions and broil for 2-3 minutes or until the cheese melts.

Serve and enjoy.

Nutritional information per serving: calories 115, total fat 9g, total carbs 2g, protein 9g

Keto Egg Muffins

Servings: 4

Ingredients

4 slices precooked bacon, crumbled

1 green onion diced

4 tablespoons shredded cheddar cheese

¼ teaspoon lemon pepper seasoning

4 eggs

Directions

Put steamer basket in your instant pot and then pour in 1 ½ cups of water in the pot.

Break the eggs in a bowl, and then season with pepper and beat well. Divide green onion, bacon and cheese evenly between 4 muffin cups. Pour the eggs into each muffin cup and stir to mix.

Place the cups onto the steamer basket. Cover and put the lid in place. Select high pressure and 8 minutes cook time. Once the timer beeps, use quick release. Open the lid carefully, remove the steamer basket with the muffin cups.

Serve the muffins immediately or keep up to a week in the

refrigerator.

Nutritional information per serving: calories 118.6, fat 8.6g, carbs 0.7g, protein 9.3g

Egg and Cheese Casserole

Servings: 5

Ingredients

1 cup whole milk

1 teaspoon pepper

1 teaspoon salt

10 eggs

2 cups shredded cheddar cheese

1 cup chopped ham

1 large onion, diced

32 ounce bag frozen hash browns, cubed

Directions

Use a non-stick cooking spray to spray the insert of an instant pot. Put a third of the hash browns at the bottom, top with a third of the onions, ham and then cheese. Repeat this two times.

Beat eggs, pepper, sat and milk in a mixing bowl until well mixed. Pour this over the layer.

Place the insert in the instant pot. Press "slow cooker", and then "Adjust" until you get to "less" adjust the time to 7 hours. If you want it to cook faster, press "slow cooker" and then adjust time to about 3-4 hours.

Once ready serve and enjoy.

Nutritional Information per serving: calories 559.3, fat 43.8g, carbs 23.4g, protein 33.8g

Breakfast Crustless Quiche

Servings: 4

Ingredients

6 eggs

1 cup shredded cheddar cheese

2 green onions, chopped

½ cup diced ham

1 cup cooked ground sausage

4 slices cooked and crumbled bacon

1/8 teaspoon ground black pepper

¼ teaspoon salt

½ cup milk

Directions

Put a trivet at the bottom of your instant pot, and then add 1 cup of water.

In a bowl, whisk together eggs, milk pepper and salt.

Add green onions, ham, sausage, bacon and cheese to a soufflé dish and mix well to incorporate everything. Pour the egg mixture into the dish and stir to mix.

Cover the dish loosely with aluminum foil and then use an aluminum foil sling to put the dish on the trivet in the instant pot.

Put the lid in place and cook for 30 minutes at manual high pressure.

Once the time elapses, use quick pressure release. Open the lid, lift the dish and remove the foil. If you want, you can sprinkle some cheese on top and broil until lightly brown.

Nutritional information per serving: calories 477.7, fat 34.9g, carbs 4.6g, protein 32.5g

Lunch Recipes

Chipotle Shredded Beef

Servings: 4-5

Ingredients

1 cup water

1 green bell pepper, seeded and cut into large chunks

1 onion, peeled and quartered

1 cup fresh cilantro, chopped roughly

1/2 teaspoon chili powder

1 teaspoon black pepper

2 teaspoons salt

2 teaspoons dried oregano

2 teaspoons dried cumin

1 tablespoon adobo sauce

1 chipotle in adobo, chopped

2 tablespoons olive oil

3 lb beef chuck roast

Directions

Season the roast with pepper and salt generously.

Press the sauté function and then add the olive oil. Brown the roast for 3-4 minutes on each side. If need be, drain the fat and return the roast back in the instant pot.

Pour the adobo sauce and the chipotle pepper over the roast and then add salt, pepper, oregano, chili powder and cumin before sprinkling the cilantro on top. Add the bell pepper and the onions and then carefully add water around the edges of the meat.

Close the Instant Pot and cook for 60 minutes at high pressure. Once the meat is done, turn allow for natural release.

Remove the meat and allow it to rest for 5 minutes. Leave the liquid in the pot as you discard the veggies. Shred the meat and then stir it into the liquid. Keep it warm until needed. You can serve with cheese taco shells.

Nutritional information per serving: calories 371.4, fat 16.5g, carbs 7.1g, protein 50.4g

Instant Pot Pork Chops

Servings: 4

Ingredients

6 ounces baby bella mushrooms, sliced

1/2 medium onion, sliced

2 tablespoons coconut oil

1/4 teaspoon cayenne pepper

1 teaspoon salt

1 teaspoon black pepper

1 teaspoon onion powder

1 teaspoon garlic powder

1 tablespoon chopped fresh parsley

1/4-1/2 teaspoon xanthan gum

1/2 cup heavy whipping cream

1 tablespoon butter

1 tablespoon paprika

4 (6-ounce) boneless pork loin chops

Directions

In a small bowl, mix the garlic powder, black pepper, paprika, cayenne pepper, onion powder and salt.

Rinse the pork chops and then pat them dry carefully. Rub 1 tablespoon of the garlic mixture into the meat. Ensure you rub both sides of the pork chops. Make sure you reserve the remaining seasonings.

In your Instant Pot, heat the coconut oil on the sauté function and then brown the prepared pork chops for 3 minutes on each side. Turn off the Instant Pot and then set the pork chops aside.

Add the onions, mushrooms and then the browned pork chops into the pot, close the lid and ensure the vent is sealed. Cook for 25 minutes on Manual High. Once done, you can release naturally. Transfer the pork chops onto a plate.

Select the sauté setting and then add the reserved seasonings, heavy cream and butter. Add 1/2 teaspoon of xanthan gum and whisk immediately.

Allow the gravy to cook for 3-5 minutes. The butter should melt and the sauce should thicken. Turn off the instant pot. Make sure when adding the xanthan gum, you add 1/4 teaspoon of the gum each time. This will allow you to test the thickness until the gravy is to your liking.

Spread the gravy over the pork chops and garnish with

parsley.

Serve the pork chops with grilled asparagus and enjoy.

Nutritional information per serving: calories 481.25, fats 32.61g, net carbs 4.06g, protein 14.75g

No Noodle Lasagna

Servings: 8

Ingredients

8 ounces mozzarella, sliced

1 jar marinara sauce (25 ounces)

1 large egg

1/2 cup Parmesan cheese

1 1/2 cups ricotta cheese

1 small onion

2 cloves garlic, minced

1 lb. ground beef

Directions

Select the sauté setting, and then brown the meat, onion and garlic.

As the meat browns, mix Parmesan and ricotta cheese in a small mixing bowl.

Add the marinara sauce into the meat, stir and then remove half of the meat sauce.

Add the mozzarella cheese to the remaining meat sauce.

Pour half the ricotta cheese mix over the mozzarella cheese and then top up with the remaining meat sauce.

Spread a layer of mozzarella cheese on top of the meat sauce. Place aside a few pieces for later.

Add the remaining ricotta cheese mixture and then layer the remaining mozzarella pieces.

Place aluminum foil over the lasagna if you wish.

Cover the pot and cook for 8-10 minutes at high pressure.

Once done, vent off the steam and carefully remove the lid. You can add any reserved cheese at this point. If you do, allow it to melt before serving.

Serve and enjoy.

Nutritional information per serving: calories 339, fat 3.2g, total carbs 6.3g, protein 36g

Low Carb Corned Beef and Cabbage

Servings: 12

Ingredients

4 celery stalks or 1 cup chopped

4 carrots or 1 cup sliced into thirds

2 onions or 1 cup sliced

1 head cabbage cut into wedges or 8 cups

2 teaspoons dried mustard

4 cloves garlic

2 teaspoons black peppercorns

6 cups water

4 pounds corned beef brisket

Directions

Put the meat into the pot and then cover it with water. Add spices into the pot, cover and select the Meat/Stew setting for 60 minutes on high.

After the time elapses, select the cancel button and then release pressure naturally for 20 minutes.

Uncover the pot, remove the meat and set aside. Add

vegetables into the pot, select "soup" function for about 15 minutes.

Once the time elapses, use quick release method, uncover, add the meat to warm through.

Serve and enjoy.

Nutritional information per serving: calories 334, total fat 22.8g, total carbs 8.1g, protein 23.7g

Dinner Recipes

Instant Pot Ribs

Servings: 6

Ingredients

5 lbs. of pork ribs

For the dry rub:

1/2 teaspoon ground coriander

1/2 teaspoon allspice

1 teaspoon paprika

1 teaspoon onion powder

1 teaspoon garlic powder

1/2 teaspoon ground black pepper

1 tablespoon erythritol or other sweetener

1 1/2 tablespoons kosher salt

For the sauce:

1/4 teaspoon xanthan gum, optional

1/2 teaspoon onion powder

1/2 tablespoon ground allspice

1/2 tablespoon ground mustard

1/4 teaspoon liquid smoke

1/2 cup water

2 tablespoons red wine vinegar

2 tablespoons erythritol or other sweetener

1/2 cup reduced sugar ketchup

Directions

Use the dry rub ingredients to season the ribs. Ensure you rub the ingredients on both sides of the ribs. Place the ribs in your Instant Pot.

In a small bowl, whisk together the water, ketchup, vinegar, liquid smoke, allspice, sweetener, onion powder and mustard. Spread the sauce mixture evenly over the ribs in the Instant Pot.

Cover the Instant Pot and ensure it is sealed properly. Select the manual setting and then cook on high pressure for 35 minutes.

After the 35 minutes, let the pressure release and then proceed to remove the lid. Place the ribs on a platter and keep them warm.

Add the xanthan gum to the sauce mixture and then select

the sauté function and cook for 10 more minutes. Once done, remove and spread the sauce over warm ribs.

Serve and enjoy.

Nutritional information for 3 ribs: calories 387, fat 29g, net carbs 2g, protein 27g

Braised Chicken Drumsticks

Servings: 6

Ingredients

1 jalapeno, halved and seeded

1/4 cup chopped cilantro, divided

1 1/2 cups jarred tomatillo sauce

1 teaspoon olive oil

1 teaspoon dried oregano

1/8 teaspoon black pepper

1 teaspoon kosher salt

1 tablespoon cider vinegar

6 chicken drumsticks, on the bone, skin removed (24 oz)

Directions

Season the chicken well with oregano, salt, pepper and vinegar and marinate it for a few hours if you have the time.

Press the sauté function and when your Instant Pot is hot, add the oil and brown both sides of the chicken. This should take about 4 minutes per side.

Add the jalapeno, tomatillo sauce and the 2 tablespoons of

cilantro and then cover your pot. Cook for 20 minutes on high pressure. This will allow the chicken to become tender.

Once done, allow the pressure to release. Remove and garnish with cilantro.

Serve and enjoy. You can serve with cauliflower rice if you wish.

Nutritional information per serving: calories 161, total fat 5g, carbs 5g, protein 22g

Instant Pot Jerk Pork Roast

Servings: 12

Ingredients

1/2 cup beef stock or broth

1 tablespoon olive oil

1/4 cup Jamaican jerk spice blend

4 lb pork shoulder

Directions

Rub the roast with the olive oil and then coat it well with the spice blend.

Select the sauté function and then brown the meat in your instant pot. Ensure you brown all the sides.

Add the beef broth into the Instant Pot, and close the lid.

Cook for 45 minutes on Manual high pressure.

Once done, release the pressure, remove and shred the meat.

Serve with your favorite veggies.

Nutritional information per serving: calories 282, fat 20g, net carbs 0g, protein 23g

Keto Chili

Servings: 10

Ingredients

1 teaspoon black pepper

2 teaspoons sea salt

1 tablespoon dried oregano

2 tablespoons cumin

1/4 cup chili powder

2 tablespoons Worcestershire sauce

1 (4-oz) can green chiles

1 (16-oz) can tomato paste

2 (15-oz) cans diced tomatoes (with liquid)

8 cloves garlic, minced

1/2 large onion, chopped

2 1/2 lbs. ground beef

1 medium bay leaf, optional

Directions

Press the sauté function, add the onion to your Instant Pot, and cook for 5-7 minutes. Add the garlic and cook for an additional minute or until fragrant.

Add the ground beef and cook it for 8-10 minutes. Use a spatula to break it apart until it is browned.

Add the rest of the ingredients except the bay leaf and stir to combine. You can place the bay leaf in the middle after you've combined the other ingredients.

Close the lid and hit the cancel button to stop the sauté function and then select the meat/stew function. This will allow the food to cook for 35 minutes.

Once done, allow for natural release or you can do a quick release if you want. If you added the bay leaf, you should remove it at this point.

Serve the chili with avocado and enjoy.

Nutritional information per serving: calories 306, total fat 18g, net carbs 10g, protein 23g

Desserts

Keto Chocolate Cheesecake

Servings: 8

Ingredients

Crust:

2 tablespoons butter melted

1 1/2 tablespoons Swerve or desired sweetener

21/2 tablespoons unsweetened cocoa powder

1/4 cup coconut flour

1/4 cup almond flour

Filling:

1 teaspoon vanilla extract

6 ounces baking chocolate melted

3/4 cup heavy cream

1/4 cup sour cream

2 large egg yolks at room temperature

1 large egg at room temperature

1/3 cup unsweetened cocoa powder

1/2 teaspoon monk fruit powder

1/2 teaspoon stevia powder

16 ounces cream cheese at room temperature

Directions

To make the crust: Place parchment paper at the bottom of a 7-inch spring form pan.

In a bowl, mix all the dry crust ingredients and then stir in the melted butter. Press the mixture into the bottom of the pan.

To make the filling: In a food processor, process the cream cheese, cocoa powder and the sweeteners. Add the egg and then the egg yolks and continue mixing.

Add in the heavy cream, sour cream, vanilla extract and melted chocolate and continue to process. Scrape the sides of the processor to mix everything.

Spread the cream cheese mixture over the crust and use a rubber spatula to smooth over the top.

Place a rack in the Instant Pot and add in 1 1/2 cups of water.

Make a sling using aluminum foil and place it over the rack. It should be long enough so that you can use it to remove the container.

Place the pan over your sling and then cover it loosely with foil. Fold the tops of the sling loosely over your cheesecake.

Cover the Instant Pot and cook for 20 minutes at high pressure. Once done, allow for natural pressure release. This should take 15 minutes.

Open the lid and lift the cheesecake out using the foil sling. Place it on a cooling rack for an hour. You can refrigerate for about 2 hours before you serve.

Serve and enjoy.

Nutritional information per serving: calories 413, total fat 38g, total carbs 13g, protein 8g

Keto Coconut Almond Cake

Servings: 8

Ingredients

Wet ingredients:

1/2 cup heavy whipping cream

1/4 cup butter, melted

2 eggs lightly whisked

Dry ingredients:

1 teaspoon apple pie spice

1 teaspoon baking powder

1/3 cup Trivia

1/2 cup unsweetened shredded coconut

1 cup almond flour

Directions

In a bowl, mix all the dry ingredients.

Add the wet ingredients one after the other and ensure you mix well as you add each ingredient.

Pour the batter into a 6-inch circular cake pan and then

cover it well with foil.

Add 2 cups of water into the Instant Pot and place a steamer rack or trivet inside. Place the pan on top.

Cook for 40 minutes at high pressure. Allow the pressure to release naturally for 10 minutes and then proceed to release the remaining pressure.

Remove the pan and allow it to cool for at least 15-20 minutes. Upend the almond cake onto a plate. Top up with almonds or coconut if you wish.

Serve and enjoy.

Nutritional information per serving: calories 326, total fat 23g, net carbs 3g, protein 5g

Keto Chocolate Mini Cakes

Servings: 2

Ingredients

1/4 cup baking cocoa

1 teaspoon vanilla extract

1/2 teaspoon baking powder

2 tablespoons heavy cream

2 large eggs

2 tablespoons splenda

Directions

In a bowl, mix all the dry ingredients.

Whisk in the wet ingredients until smooth.

Spray the ramekins with cooking spray and fill each ramekin halfway with the batter.

Add a cup of water to the Instant Pot and put the trivet inside.

Carefully place the ramekins on top of the trivet and place the lid. Ensure that the valve is closed.

Cook for 9 minutes on Manual high pressure.

After the beep, do a quick release and then remove the mini cakes and flip them onto a plate.

Nutritional information per serving: calories 168, fat 9g, carbohydrates 7g, protein 9g

Ricotta Lemon Cheesecake

Servings: 6

Ingredients

For batter:

2 eggs

1/2 teaspoon lemon extract

Lemon juice from one lemon

Zest of one lemon

1/3 cup ricotta cheese

1/4 cup Truvia

8 oz cream cheese

For topping:

1 teaspoon Truvia

2 tablespoons sour cream

Directions

Mix all the ingredients except the eggs until smooth. You can use a stand mixer to mix. Check the sweetness and adjust if you wish.

Add the eggs and mix again to incorporate them. Don't over-beat the eggs as this could make the crust break.

Pour the batter into a 6-inch greased spring-form pan and cover with a silicon lid or foil.

Add 2 cups of water in the Instant Pot and place the trivet inside. Place the greased pan on top of the trivet.

Cook for 30 minutes on high pressure and then allow for natural release.

Mix the toppings, spread over the cake and then place the cake in the refrigerator for 6-8 hours.

Serve and enjoy.

Nutritional information per serving: calories 181, fat 16g, carbs 2g, protein 5g

Low Carb Cheesecake

Servings: 8

Ingredients

Top layer:

2 teaspoons granulated swerve

1/2 cup sour cream or Greek yogurt full-fat

Filling:

1/4 cup heavy whipping cream

3 eggs, room temperature

Zest of 1 small lemon

1 teaspoon fresh orange zest

1/2 teaspoon vanilla extract

1/2 cup + 2 tablespoons granulated swerve

16 oz cream cheese, room temperature

Directions

Line a 6-inch or 7-inch spring form pan or push pan with parchment paper and then oil the bottom of the pan very lightly. Ensure that the parchment paper is taller than the pan by at least 2 inches. Wrap some foil round at the bottom of the prepared pan. This will prevent water from getting into the cheesecake. It will also stop the cake from seeping out of your pan. Once you have prepared the pan, set it aside.

Use a hand-held mixer or a stand mixer to mix Swerve, orange peels, cream cheese, heavy cream, lemon and vanilla until smooth.

Add in the eggs one at a time and then mix gently until just combined. You should not over mix. If you do, the cheesecake will turn out lumpy instead of creamy.

Gently pour the batter into your prepared pan and then place a paper towel over it. Wrap a piece of foil over it to hold it in place. This is why you should ensure that the piece of foil you placed on the pan is taller than the pan. This way, you can just fold it or pinch it in to hold the paper towel in place.

Add 1 1/2 cups of water to your inner liner pot and then place the trivet inside.

Create a foil sling and then put the cheesecake pan at the center of it and lower it onto the trivet. Remember to leave the foil sling inside.

Place the lid on the Instant Pot and ensure that you set the valve to 'sealing'. Cook for 37 minutes on manual.

In the meantime, prepare the topping by mixing the topping ingredients, and then set aside.

Once the cooking time is over, allow for natural pressure release. This should take 18 minutes. Once the time is up, open the valve and carefully remove the lid once all the pressure is released.

Use the foil sling to lift the cheesecake from your Instant Pot. If there's liquid on top of the cheesecake, you can dab it off using a paper towel.

Spread the topping over the hot cheesecake and then replace the foil or paper towel on the cheesecake. Proceed to refrigerate for at least 8 hours.

Remove and serve chilled.

Nutritional information per serving: fat 23.8g, protein 6.8g, net carbs 3g

I need your help...

We have come to the end of the book. Thank you for reading and congratulations for reading until the end.

If you found the book valuable, can you recommend it to others? One way to do that is to post a review on Amazon.

If you have any questions or problems, please contact us: hello@freedomdestination.com

Thank you and good luck!

Bonus: Subscribe To The Free Weight Loss Report

When you subscribe to Freedom Destination via email, you will get free access to an ebook. All you have to do is enter your email address to get instant access.

The Introduction Manual is more than just an introduction to the diet. Instead, it discusses the science behind how we gain and lose weight as well as what absolutely needs to be done to attack that stubborn body fat that, until now, has been so challenging to get rid of.

Here are the preview of what you'll get:

- Rapid Weight Loss
- How This System Works
- Why This Diet
- Why 3 Weeks?
- 21 Days To Make A Habit
- Fat Loss VS. Weight Loss
- Nutrients

- Protein, Fat, Carbohydrates

- The Food Pyramid And Obesity

- Fiber

- Metabolism

- How We Get Fat

- Triglycerides

- How To Get Thin

- Diet Overview

- Meal Frequency

- Water

- Diet Essentials

- Let's Get Started

You can access it here: http://bit.ly/2tUb9cp